Eat Nourish And Grow

Live Healthy, Grow Better & Lose Weight

By
Cheryl Barnhart

Cheryl Barnhart

ACKNOWLEDGMENTS

For my students and friends, who all
selflessly helped me in writing this book.
Special thanks to those who asked, insisted
and assisted me in turning the seminars in
this practical form. All Rights Reserved
2012-2015 @ Cheryl Barnhart

TABLE OF CONTENTS

Chapter 3 - Understanding the 5 W's Of Eat Nourish and Grow

- What
- Who
- When
- Where
- Whom

Chapter 4 - Process to Reach a Healthy Point in Life

- Immediate Process
- Quick Process
- Slow Process

Chapter 5 - Telling the World Why Eating Healthy Is Important

- Children
- Youth
- Adult
- Elderly

Chapter 6 - Make Sure You Always Talk With Full Understanding

- **Be a Doer of What You Say**
- **Stay Confident In All That You Say**

Chapter 7 - Selecting the Right Foods for Your Health Needs

- **Hepatitis B**
- **High Blood Pressure**
- **Obesity**
- **Skin Irritation Issues**
- **Perfect Eyesight**

Chapter 8 - Losing Weight Even As You Stay Healthy

- **Stay Choosy With What You Eat**
- **Make Sure You Never Eat Things That Will Cause More Harm To You**
- **Enjoy the Healthy Foods You Eat**

Chapter 9 - Get Your Children Involved In the Eating Healthy Process

- **Try To Make Healthy Cookies with Honey At Home for Them**
- **Make Sure Fruit Juices Are Blended Home For Them**
- **Inculcate The Different Vegetables In The Foods They Eat.**
- **Do Not Fight Them to Eat Healthy Foods Because Convincing Children Can Be Quite Hard**
- **Take the Steps Below Seriously To Get Them into the Process**
- **Create a Food Schedule with Them**
- **Make Sure You Eat Exactly What They Eat**
- **Make Sure You Have a Three Bite Rule Set Up**
- **Involve Your Children in the Shopping Process for the Healthy Foods You Buy**
- **Have a List of All the Foods They Love and Those They Hate**
- **Cook Meals Together**

- Have a Lot of Fun

Chapter 10 - Eating Healthy Even During Holidays

- Be Cautious How You Eat During Holidays
- Some Recommended Foods That Will Keep You Healthier During Holidays
- Staying Healthy Tips All Through Holidays

Chapter 11 - Acquire More Information on the Internet about Eating Healthy

- Use the Internet to Research
- Ask Others Who Have More Knowledge in the Area
- Understand What the Different Foods Can Help You Get

Chapter 12 - Never Forget To Involve Exercising

- Regular Exercises Are Important
- Make Sure You Have a Weekly Exercise Timetable
- Always Start the Workout Process Slowly
- Simple Workout Techniques Are Best

Chapter 13 - Drink More and More Water

- Drinking Clean Water Is the Key

Chapter 14 - Stay Away From Junk Foods

- Buying Junk Foods Will Only Cost You Money and Your Health
- Do You Know How The Food Is Prepared?
- Cook and Pack For In Lunch Boxes to the Office

INTRODUCTION

A lot of people tend to believe that their aim to lose weight means they are living a good and healthy lifestyle. Weight loss although being a difficult process doesn't mean you are living a healthy life if you proceed with it. Being obese is not a good thing; however, you should never settle for weight loss to be the best way out.

This Book, however, is being written to give you the best value for information and also explain to you the reasons you need to stay healthy. Staying healthy really involves three things, eating healthy, staying nourished and growing. When you are able to eat well, you are always in perfect state or shape, which means you grow very well and healthy. A lot of people eat food in moderation but still gain lots of weights. This goes to show that living and staying healthy has nothing to do with losing weight.

Weight loss is a chapter on its own, which will be tackled in subsequent pages as you read on. However, you need to try generally your best to eat healthy so that you do not have any issues with your health as you grow. This

Book will be the eye opener you have always wished for. So, take your time to read every page and make sure you try your best to be motivated enough to go through with the different procedures and recommendations are given in this Book, that is if it falls within what you believe.

CHAPTER 1
Understanding The Importance Of Nutrition

There are so many things that come together to explain the world of nutrition. Most people feel they have all the nutrients they need because they eat the very best of meals with highly tasty seasonings used to make them. Well, being nourished is different from nutrition, which is one thing you need to understand. Today, the food industry has messed up almost everything good that we used to have with food. This doesn't mean there aren't good foods that are free from chemical additives you can eat to stay healthy.

Nutrition involves a lot, but buying and cooking your own meals helps to bring all of these together. A lot of families prefer to eat originally made foods that are not processed. However, not every family can afford to buy them.

a) To help you stand out from your colleagues

When you are nurtured, you tend to look healthy. Staying healthy can give you a refined and younger look, which means you will always have a better stand for promotions. In big companies, there are so many factors that are considered before promotions are given. Having a healthy look and looking stronger is one of the best standards that most companies give their workers promotions on.

b) To keep you very strong

Eating highly nutritional foods help to give you the strength you need to go about your day to day activities.

c) To make it easy for you to participate in every and any activity

When you eat well, and you are strong, you are able to have fun with your children as you involve yourself in every activity they are involved in. This makes them happy and keeps the family together.

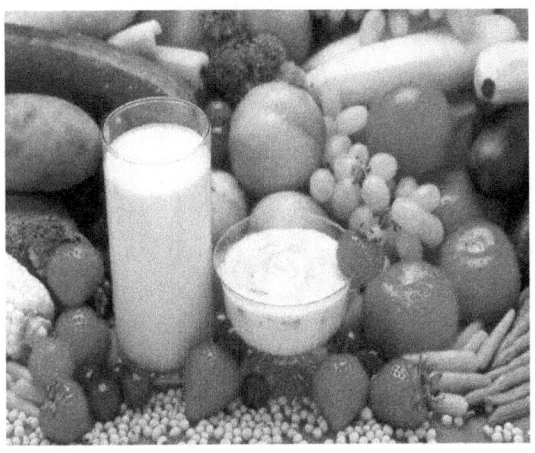

CHAPTER 2
What Are Eat, Nourish, And Grow?

The three words Eat, Nourish and Grow have unique meanings that when you understand will help you know exactly what you need to do in having a healthy eating life.

Understanding The Word 'Eat.'

The word 'Eat' means a lot if you believe staying healthy can give you a better life. Eating doesn't mean you should eat just about anything that you see or feel like eating. Before you eat, it is important to look at the food before you and decide if it is something, you will really want to have in your system. Many people try to do away with the thought of health when they eat. However, eating foods that contain a lot of fats will eventually kill you. Life is the most important asset we have. This is why we should always work at staying healthier and stronger especially through the foods we eat.

Understanding The Word 'Nourish.'

The word 'Nourish' can affect our lives in so many different ways. Eating nourishing meals means eating meals that are well balanced. Preparing balanced meals can be very difficult which is why you need to try your very best to have a well-planned food preparation process to meet the level of balanced meals.

Understanding The Word 'Grow.'

The word 'Grow' can be also applied in different settings. For instance, a lot of people realizing that eating healthy foods makes they grow better have decided to grow their own food by having backyard gardens or farms. This is an amazing decision or action. However, it needs to be tackled with so much care.

If you have made the decision to feed your family with healthy and safe foods that used to be in existence some years ago, then you will definitely need to produce them on your own. You will still need to be cautious about the seeds that you use for growing your food. When you order or buy soybean, corn or any other seeds to plant in your vegetable garden, make sure the seeds you buy are not genetically made or engineered. You can find original and natural seeds that are not genetically engineered to buy.

When you are able to find a good retailer of original and natural seeds, you can buy as many seeds as possible and be assured of having great value for money when they grow and you feed your family with natural foods.

Staying True To Yourself

In the world of healthy living and eating, all you have is to stay true to yourself. A lot of people try to act all healthy and nutritious when they are with friends, but eat junk foods when they are alone. Doing this doesn't mean a thing especially since all you will be achieving is to kill yourself and do yourself more harm than good. The first discipline to live a life free from health issues is to be true to you. When you stay true to yourself, it takes off unnecessary pressure from you, and you are able to understand how human you are and that you can make mistakes.

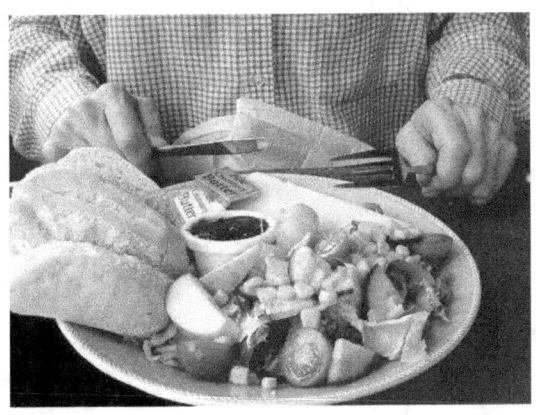

CHAPTER 3
Understanding The 5 W's Of Eat Nourish And Grow

Understanding what, whom, when, where and whom where 'Eat Nourish, and Grow' is concerned can be quite complicated. This is one of the reasons you need to understand these 5 W's to obtain a deeper meaning into this way of life.

WHAT

So, what does it mean for me to eat, nourish and grow? If you value your life and do not want to end up in a sick bed anytime soon, you will want to live a healthy eating life. There are so many foods that we eat in huge amounts that cause us much harm. You can eat any kind of food you want. However, eating in moderation as well as eating more healthy foods helps to keep you on the safer side.

WHO

Who should eat healthily? A lot of people think they do not need to eat healthy because they look fine and are always working out. Well, although working out is amazing and great, you need to make it a must to eat lots of healthy foods. No matter how strong and healthy you see yourself, you need to eat healthy in order to be in tiptop shape at all times.

WHEN

When do I have to maintain a healthy diet? It is funny when many people have to wait to fall seriously ill before they decide to maintain a healthy diet. Maintaining a healthy diet and eating well should start from now. Procrastination, where your eating habits are concerned, will only do you a lot of harms. There is no special time to start maintaining a healthy diet, but the ideal time is now.

WHERE

Where do I buy naturally grown foods from? If you have decided to have a healthy diet and eat only naturally made foods without excessive chemical additives, you have more work to do. Although making this decision is wonderful, you will need to be very careful how you go about finding the right and safe foods to buy. There are so many online and offline food stores that advertise selling foods grown with no chemicals. Well, it is and will always be up to you to decide which shopping center will do and which one to trust to offer you the safe foods you desire.

WHOM

Whom do I go to for advice regarding how to plan my eating life? Today, there are so many health experts who have a high level of understanding and vast experience where eating right is concerned. You can visit a nutritionist to help you plan your eating life and also recommend some foods that will work perfectly for you. This will do you a lot of good.

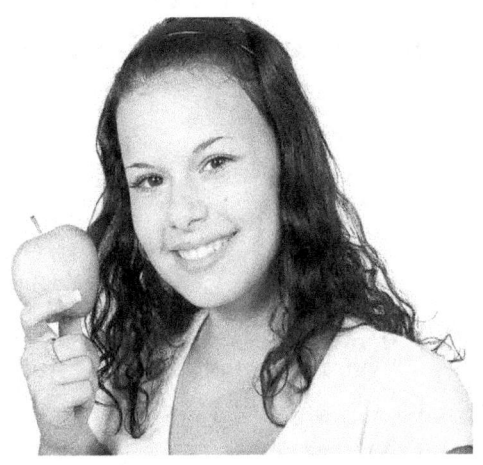

CHAPTER 4
Process To Reach A Healthy Point In Life

In life, there are processes that need to be taken seriously. However, most people do not realize that every decision they take in their lives follows a process. The more you understand this, the better life gets for you.

Immediate Process

Reaching a healthy point in life can be done as soon as now. Yes, you can make the decision today, and you can decide to stick to it forever. This is mostly recommended for people who are bedridden and have serious health issues that need them to change their diet immediately or as soon as possible. You should never wish to reach this point in life before you move on the healthy dieting way.

Quick Process

The quick process of reaching a healthy point in life mostly has to do with people who realize they are reaching a high level of unhealthy living and rectify their mistakes before things reach a level they cannot control. The quick process involves an individual searching for the best ways to stay healthy all round.

Slow Process

The slow process involves people take some time to come to the realization that they need help. Most people due to the high level of the activities they do think they are in tip top shape. Well, these kinds of people find it difficult to embrace the idea of eating and staying healthy like others who realize they truly need help do. So, they take the process slowly and do not attack it with the aggressiveness that they need to.

CHAPTER 5
Telling The World Why Eating Healthy Is Important

When you are able to understand better what eating healthy is all about and also how important it is to eat the right foods, the right way; you will always want to tell the world about it. When you feel free from chemical foods and other diseases, you will always want the world to share in your joy.

CHILDREN

Speaking to children about healthy eating can be quite tricky. This is because children do not really care about the health speeches they hear when they are now growing. All a child will mostly want is for his or her parents to buy the best chocolates and candies on a daily basis for them. Although parents should understand that it is good to make their children feel loved, there are other ways to make your children understand that eating too many sweets is harmful to them. Depending on your child and how they reason or how they behave, there are different approaches that can be used to get them to understand better the uniqueness and importance of healthy eating.

YOUTH

Where the youth is concerned, getting messages across to them especially where healthy eating is concerned is actually quite easy. This is because both male and female teenagers have over the years started to care a lot about their look. Most girls do not want to be overweight or gain more than a specific size, which goes the same for the guys too. This is why telling them the right foods to eat, how to eat when to eat and also what to eat always sinks in for most of them.

ADULT

Most adults rely more on health supplements to give all they need. Although this has proven to work for most of them, it is always important for adults to be advised on how they can eat right from the meals they eat so that they do not have to spend so much money on costly health supplements. At a certain age health supplements help a lot, but during your ages of 35 to 45, you should still be able to work at maintaining a healthy diet for a healthier life on your own without any such help from supplements. You can take vitamin C tablets to improve your metabolism and help you with strength from day to day or cod liver oil to help nourish your skin from inside out.

ELDERLY

For the elderly, taking health supplements is mostly a normal thing although not all elderly men and women take them. If you want to speak to the elderly to alter the way they eat, there are so many ways to do that. Due to the fact that the elderly know right from wrong and have come a long way in life, talking to them to make a switch and eat healthier is easier. So, just try to be friendly and give them some clear cut recommendations of what to eat and they will perhaps do what you say.

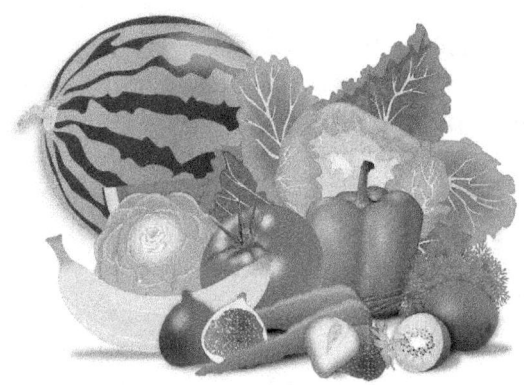

CHAPTER 6
Make Sure You Always Talk With Full Understanding

If you have benefited from living a healthier life and eating the right way, make sure you still research to know more before you advise people. You need to understand that making some recommendations of foods can be bad for one person although good for another due to different body types and systems as well as allergic issues. So, make sure you never recommend foods or health products to people as you advise them to eat nutritious food. Make sure you just tell them your story, and that will do the magic for you.

Be A Doer Of What You Say

So, you are telling people to eat healthy foods and eat more vegetables as well. However, do you do the same? Yes, a lot of people who advise people on eating healthy foods are the worst where eating healthy is concerned. Make sure you do not just open your mouth and talk because you have researched and knew. Do what you tell others to do and you will find fulfillment in yourself.

Stay Confident In All That You Say

When you practice what you are teaching, it becomes very easy for you to speak with all the confidence you need. Also, you are able to learn more as you educate others more. If you do not speak with confidence to people about eating nutritious foods and staying healthy, they will never take you seriously.

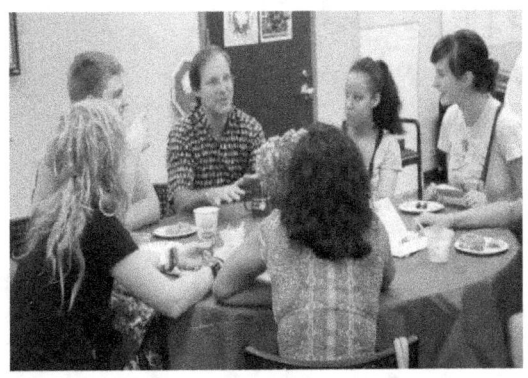

CHAPTER 7
Selecting The Right Foods For Your Health Needs

Below are some few health issues that people face on a daily basis all over the world. Under every health issue, some general recommendations will be made to give you an idea what you need to do in staying away from these health issues and how to maintain the best health even as you deal with these problems. Knowing the right foods to eat can help take you out of or take you away from ill health. However, if you have to deal with some illnesses or diseases already, eating the right foods can repair your system, heal and sustain you.

Type 2 Diabetes

When you have to deal with Type 2 Diabetes, you will need to think more about controlling your blood sugar through your meals. A very important part of controlling diabetes is to make sure you eat the right foods with the right serving sizes. If you know very well the number of servings of each food to eat, and you make sure the right servings are eaten, you are then able to eat balanced diets, which help to keep your blood sugar level at the right point.

There is no doubt however that, eating the right food serving sizes can be quite challenging. Over the past years, the sizes of servings have increased. This means you might not be able to eat all the food that is served to you. When you are however able to know these portions very well, you can decide exactly how much you have to eat and how much you should not. Below are some portions that you can consider in order to determine the right servings for you:

- Some years ago, a plate of French fries was about 2.4 ounces and came with 210 calories per serving. However, it is not the same today. Today, a plate of French fries has 610 calories and weight 6.9 ounces.

- Some years ago, 2 slices of pepperoni pizza contained 500 calories. However, today the same 2 slices have 850 calories.
- Soda drinks some years back came in 6.5-ounce bottles and had 85 calories. It, however, is not the same today. It comes in 20-ounce bottles with 250 calories.

There more and more examples that can be given. However, the few above should show you how things have changed over the years. This is what has led to making it difficult for so many people to live a healthier eating life. However, it is not impossible. Although it might seem difficult, you can decide to have a free life free from the thought that you even have to deal with Type 2 Diabetes. All you need to do is to be serious about apportioning your servings very well and knowing what to eat at what time and how much to eat at any given period. You can make the right diet changes to your daily life, which can help reduce your weight and also the level of your blood sugar. Just be patient and make sure you do not tire yourself out.

High Blood Pressure

It isn't surprising that so many doctors are always ready to prescribe medications for people with hypertension health conditions also known as High Blood Pressure. This being said does not mean that medications are not good or should not be taken especially if prescribed by expert health practitioners. However, it is high time that the many natural methods of reducing high blood pressure are introduced to patients all over the world. These natural methods are fulfilling than any other chemical prescriptions because most of the medications come with side effects while the natural methods do not have any side effects whatsoever.

It has been proven that healthy diets that contain high levels of magnesium, calcium and potassium have a unique way of reducing and aiding to control hypertension. Also, healthy diet for such patients should have a reasonable amount of fatty acids, but very little salt, saturated fats, and sugar. Below are some foods you should always have your meals for complete health and relief from the pressure this health issue comes with.

- **Sunflower Seeds** – These seeds come rich in magnesium, potassium, and phytosterols. These can help in reducing the level of cholesterol in your system, which is great. This is because high cholesterol levels can cause your arteries and blood vessels to become narrow which will in turn raise your blood pressure.

- **Spinach** – Spinach is also rich in magnesium and folate. It helps in preventing heart diseases. The folate that spinach has helped in protecting the body from homocysteine. Homocysteine, when produced in excess in the body, can lead to strokes and heart attacks. When you use spinach in meals, however, make sure you cook it very little. It is mostly better to eat while it is raw and not touched with heat.

- **Garlic** – Garlic is also an amazing food that helps to thin the blood and makes sure blood vessel clogs never happen, which reduces the pressure of blood. You can chew a clove or two of garlic every day. However, due to its smell it will be better if you take it in supplement forms.

- **Broccoli** – Broccoli is a vegetable filled with lots of nutrition. It is high in potassium and chromium. Chromium in broccoli helps in regulating insulin and blood sugar. However, make sure you do not overcook it in order to retain more of its nutrients. Steaming it is better recommended than boiling or even eats raw.

There are so many other foods that you can eat like hawthorn, fish that contains omega 3, bananas, tomatoes, etc.

OBESITY

Being obese is not a good thing. This is why a lot of people try their very best to stay in shape. However, with so many things going on in our daily lives, it can become very difficult to live in tip top shape. This is why if you are obese, you are possibly not to be blamed. Most people realize they are obese when it is too late while others walk themselves right into it because of some problems they were facing. Below are some foods to eat and also some tips on how to get rid of obesity in a reasonable time:

- You need always to know that, working on weight loss is not an easy process especially when you have grown to love and appreciate all those bad foods that made you obese.

- Make sure you stayed focused and prepared to take the process very seriously. Being determined helps to make the process faster than it would normally be.

- Make sure you have a regular workout session. You can decide to take long walks every morning or jogging can also be perfect. All you need to do is to work out to burn excess fat as well as keep you in the perfect shape.

- Some foods you need to eat include vegetables (cabbages, carrots, spinach, tomatoes, garlic, lettuce, broccoli, etc.), unrefined sugar specifically brown sugar, brown rice instead of white rice, brown bread, etc.

- Drinking freshly made lemon juice from your own kitchen on a daily basis also helps.

- You can treat yourself to something unhealthy once or twice every month. This will depend on how strong you are not to go back.

Skin Irritation Issues

Dry seasons have a high tendency of reducing the beauty of your skin by making it look very dry. Using creams and moisturizers can work, however, it is always better to make sure your skin looks great the natural way. Skin irritations will be a thing of the past if you know the right foods to eat and also how to take very good care of yourself. Below are some foods that you can eat to prevent skin irritations and help give you the perfect skin you have always wished for.

- **Beet-Root** – This food is not only delicious. However, it can help you look very young and have a fresh skin for so many years. Eating beetroot regularly helps to brighten your skin. Although a lot of people find it difficult to eat beetroot, it is easier to eat when you boil in hot water or eat with freshly squeezed lemon juice.

- **Indian Gooseberry** – This food is also good in vitamin A, which helps in the production of collagen that is needed to retain the shine of your skin. To see the effectiveness of Indian gooseberry, you should eat it every morning when you haven't eaten anything. Collagen degeneration is prevented when you eat Indian gooseberry, and it allows your body to increase the production of collagen to a greater extent.

- **Lemon Juice Or Fruit** – Lemon is a fruit that helps you get rid of many skin irritation issues. It comes rich in vitamin C, which is another good nutrient, which helps in high collagen production. All you need to do is to squeeze some small lemon juice into a cup or glass of hot water and drink it every morning. This should be done on a daily basis. It can also be done in the evening before you go to bed.

- **Tomatoes** – Tomatoes are rich in lycopene, which is an anti-ageing agent. Also, lycopene stops the occurrence of the harm the sun rays cause to the skin. The more you eat tomatoes, the more lycopene you get which also helps to prevent pimples on your face and other parts of your skin. You can blend it or chew it raw to increase your skin's glow.

Some other foods you should eat include sweet potatoes, apples, strawberries, etc.

Perfect Eyesight

Your aim to have perfect eyesight is never in vain. A lot of people lie to themselves by saying that poor vision is inevitable and also a very normal part of aging. Well, never believe what they say because it is all not true. The human body was made to be its own healing machine. This is why with the right foods; you can get the right cells in your body to work in improving your eyesight. Apart from the right foods, eye exercises help in strengthening all eye muscles that are weakened.

When you give your eyes, the right nutritional aid needed, you help them to see better and stronger.

- Eating carrots or blending carrots to drink as the juice helps to prevent eyesight issues and improves eyesight considerably. Carrots contain beta carotene, which benefits your eyes in huge proportions.

- Stay away from taking in a lot of coffee or tea.

- Make sure you do not smoke as well.

- Reduce your intake on sugary stuff as well as junk foods.

- Other foods you should regularly eat includethe lean chicken, mango juice, fish, spinach, turkey, broccoli, tomatoes, etc.

- Make sure you take in more vegetable blended juices from time to time.

Cheryl Barnhart

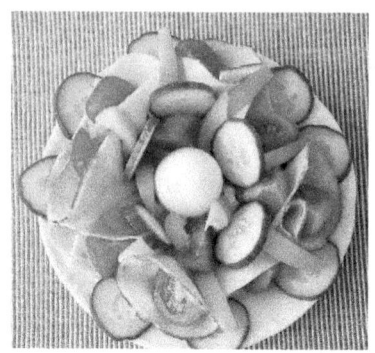

CHAPTER 8
Losing Weight Even As You Stay Healthy

If you have decided to lose some weight for whatever reason, it is important first to understand it is a good step in the right direction. However, weight loss has over the years become a different thing altogether where people involve themselves in habits they should not, just because they are desperate. The fact that you want to lose weight does not mean you should forget your health. Being healthy and strong is worth more than losing many pounds when you are weak and unhealthy.

Stay Choosy With What You Eat

To begin with, make sure you are always selective with the foods that you eat. Generally, eating too much of saturated fats and refined sugars is never the best. This is why you should be very careful with the specific foods that you eat and also why you eat what you eat. Although it might seem too technical, it will be better to know what nutrients you are getting from every foodgroup you put into your mouth. This is one unique way to stay focused and to always have your health in mind even as you eat to lose weight.

Make Sure You Never Eat Things That Will Cause More Harm To You

Every individual has urges and cravings for specific foods. The fact that you have cravings for a specific unhealthy food does not mean you should eat it. Most times, you will eat that food and later regret you did. This is why you should be disciplined and always tries to stay focused with what you do. This does not mean you should starve yourself. It is important to eat. However, make sure you eat smaller chunks of healthy foods all through the day.

Enjoy The Healthy Foods You Eat

You should try your very best to enjoy the healthy foods that you eat. It is true that some healthy foods can be quite irritating to eat because they are tasteless. However, there are so many recipes that are available for you to use in making sumptuous meals out of the vegetables and other healthy foods you hate to eat.

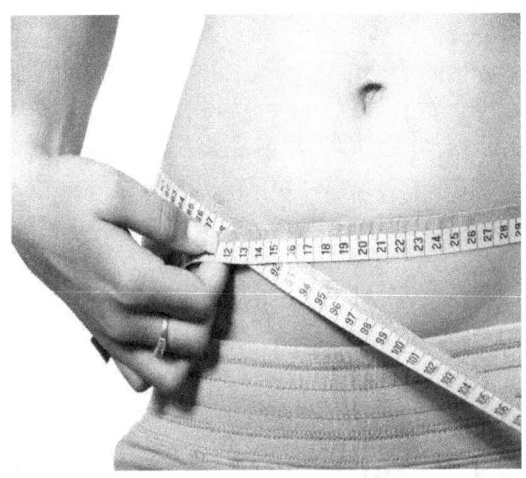

CHAPTER 9
Get Your Children Involved In
The Eating Healthy Process

Although children are adorable, they can be very difficult from time to time especially when they want to have their way. This does not mean they cannot be swayed by love and some pampering to go the way you want. Depending on the child involved, the process can be very easy or difficult. Some parents prefer to make meals and add all the things they want their children to eat without letting them know while others get them involved. Depending on the child involved, you decide which will work best for your situation.

Try To Make Healthy Cookies With Honey At Home For Them

You can always benefit from the many healthy cookie recipes available online made with honey for your children.

Yes, honey is used in place of white or even brown sugar, which makes it healthier. You will realize that these cookies taste even better than the normal cookies that the children are used to.

Make Sure Fruit Juices Are Blended Home For Them

Giving your children fruit juices every day is an amazing way to keep them healthy. However, you need to ensure all juices are made in your home and from your kitchen. This way, you are able to make them with all the love and the best of fruits to achieve high level of nutritional value.

Inculcate The Different Vegetables In The Foods They Eat

Make sure you do your best to convince them to eat vegetables raw. You can promise them gifts or time in the park when they eat these vegetables. It always works, and as time goes on, they will get used to these vegetables.

Do Not Fight Them To Eat Healthy Foods Because Convincing Children Can Be Quite Hard

Never try to fight or abuse your children verbally when they do not eat vegetables like you want. Doing this will only make, they feel like you do not like them and will make them hate the vegetables more. Try your best to convince them. Get to know the soft spot of your child and use it to get him or her to eat the vegetables.

Take The Steps Below Seriously To Get Them Into The Process

- **Create A Food Schedule With Them**

Children love routines, and they also love to create their own lists and schedules. So, make sure weekly food schedules are made with them with only a few rules. For instance, they will need to promise to eat one vegetable and one fruit in two meals every day. This works like magic; you can try it.

- **Make Sure You Eat Exactly What They Eat**

Children are very exciting but are smart too. When you tell your children to eat one thing while you eat another thing, the level of trust starts to break from there. Make sure you eat the same things you give your child to consume. You can dine on other things later in your room, but make sure you eat with them so that they feel safe and motivated.

- **Make Sure You Have A Three Bite Rule Set Up**

So many kids hate broccoli. So, do not be worked up if your child clearly hates it. Just try your best to introduce a three bite rule. If your child hates it after three bites, take it out of the meal so that they can finish up.

- **Involve Your Children In The Shopping Process For The Healthy Foods You Buy**

When you take your children along with you for shopping, they get to understand where what they eat comes from. This makes them excited to eat more.

- **Have A List Of All The Foods They Love And Those They Hate**

Make sure you know all the foods they love and those they hate. Introduce those they love with those they hate and make them eat them together little by little. They will definitely start to love some of those they dislike.

- **Cook Meals Together**

After shopping, make sure you cook together with them. When children help with cooking, they are happy and feel it is their obligation to eat what they helped cook.

- **Have A Lot Of Fun**

From time to time, you should let your children eat some ice creams and chocolates for a treat. This will make them happy, and that is how it is supposed to be. Do not be too harsh on them.

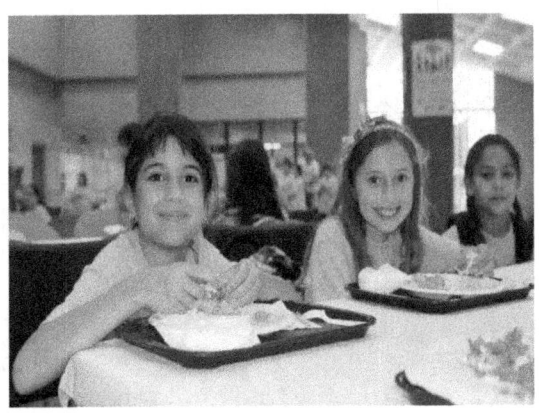

CHAPTER 10
Eating Healthy Even During Holidays

Although many people find it fulfilling to live a healthy dieting life, there are specific times when things can really get out of hand. Yes, holidays have been known to present a great challenge to people on healthy diets all over the world. This is why you need to be cautious and make sure you do not fall to this holiday breaking syndrome. Although no one is saying you should not eat the things you love, you should make sure you stay healthy when you eat these things by eating them in moderation or replacing them with healthier alternatives. There are times when you have no control over the situation especially when you are at a dinner where you need to eat something. This doesn't mean that you should eat in excess.

Be Cautious How You Eat During Holidays

The most important thing to be cautious about while holidays is what you eat into your system. Do not be blinded by those who eat just anything and mess up the long hours and days you have put into keeping your health on point. Make sure you have the right foods prepared at home and eat them even before you step out for the occasions you go to. This will fill your tummy and make it difficult for you to eat more when you go out.

Some Recommended Foods That Will Keep You Healthier During Holidays

- Dark leafy veggies like dark lettuces, spinach, kale, and others will be perfect. Kale, for instance, is a veggie that a lot of people do not love to eat; however, it is amazing and can be tasty depending on the recipe used.

Make sure you use only oil and vinegar for your salad dressings. Do not entertain creamy dressings.

- Grapes and grapefruit juice. Although you will come into contact with different grape juices and also grape wines, make sure you do not over-indulge. Just be cautious and take some few sips if possible.

- Berries come with high levels of vitamin C and also fiber. This makes them the best fruits to have at home and even in your car during the holidays.

- Beans can be another amazing food for you during the holidays. They have a lot of fiber that helps to fill your tummy and prevents you from getting hungry easily. So, eating bean salads, for instance, will help prevent eating more than you should.

Other foods that you should never take for granted all through the holidays and after the holidays include tomatoes, cabbages, Brussels sprouts, broccoli, garlic, green tea, and others.

Staying Healthy Tips All Through Holidays

- Make sure you have a quick snack of your healthy foods before you go out to any program or event. This will help make you full and help you make the right choices with the things you eat when you are at the event.

- If you have meat served at a party or family dinner, but you do not want to eat meat, eat only the veggies and bread or grains.

- Make sure you sleep very well before you go out for a program or an event. This will keep you relaxed and prevent you from making hasty decisions about food that you can regret.

- Go out for long walks to burn some calories and also get some fresh air.

- Make sure you use your spare time to look for new healthy food recipes that you can make at home.

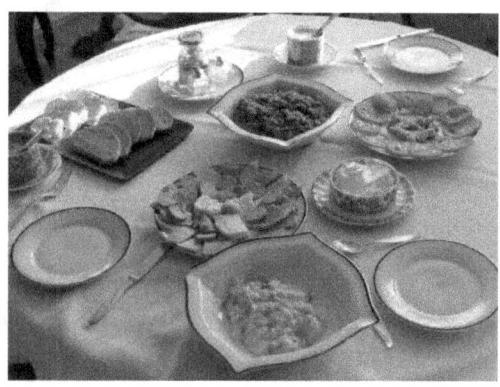

CHAPTER 11
Acquire More Information On The Internet About Eating Healthy

With the internet, obtaining information today has become very easy. A lot of people do not understand why they should search the internet for information. The truth, however, is that online information has a unique way of giving you the true feel of what you should do. Although there are so many ways you can find the best eating healthy tips and other recipes, you need to try your best to find sources that are credible.

Use The Internet To Research

Although the internet is the best place to source out as much information as possible, you might end up having problems if you do not use the right sources. Although the internet is a good place for information, not every source is credible nor has the right solutions or answers to your questions. This is why you need to research and try your very best to only read Books that are from credible sources and sites that give you the best information.

Ask Others Who Have More Knowledge In The Area

In every field of study and every area of life, there are so many people who have advanced knowledge and can help you out. This is why you need to be very careful and cautious in getting the right information from experts who are more knowledgeable than you are. Not all experts will recommend or follow the theories you have. This is why you need to take the process of soaking in information about healthy dieting and eating cautiously.

Understand What The Different Foods Can Help You Get

Also, it is important for you to find out about the different health foods available in the system and the different vitamins and nutrients they come with. Knowing this will help you plan your diet very well. It will also help you decide which foods are the best for you and which ones are not.

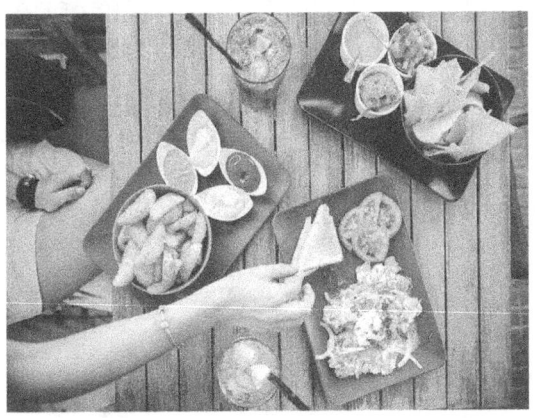

CHAPTER 12
Never Forget To Involve Exercising

Staying healthy has a lot also to do with exercises. Never think that you can eat your way to staying healthy and strong. Make sure you have some form of workout routine or schedule in place to back it up.

Regular Exercises Are Important

Regular workouts help a lot. If you do not believe in the power of workouts, it is time to start to believe in it. Workouts like running, jogging, and long walks have proven to work magic in helping you stay in the best shape.

Make Sure You Have A Weekly Exercise Timetable

Do not make the workout process to be a burden. Make sure you have routine and specific days to exercise every week. This will help you stay focused.

Always Start The Workout Process Slowly

If you want to get into vigorous workouts, there will be the need for you always to think of starting slowly. Starting slowly will help you a lot to get used to the workout process.

Simple Workout Techniques Are Best

Also, try your best to stay away from workout routines that are too complicated and up above you. Stick to the simple workout methods you know for your own good.

CHAPTER 13
Drink More And More Water

Instead of drinking more wine and other carbonated drinks, it will be better for you to drink more water. Drinking more water helps to clear your system and get rid of all unwanted toxins in your system. The more water you drink, the better your health gets.

Drinking Clean Water Is The Key

You should make it a must to drink at least 8 glasses of clean water every day. Drinking untreated water can be dangerous to your health. So, make sure you take your health seriously.

Eat Nourish And Grow

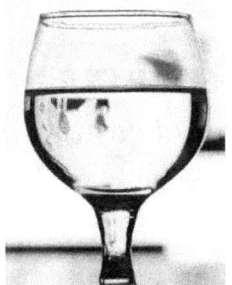

CHAPTER 14
Stay Away From Junk Foods

Buying Junk Foods Will Only Cost You Money And Your Health

A lot of people are addicted to junk foods because they do not have to make them on their own and because junk foods are very tasty. The truth, however, is that they are simply unhealthy and will be harmful to your health no matter how tasty they are. This is why you should never be blinded by their cheap pricing and lovely taste. All you need to think of is saving your life and by doing so; there will be the need for you to stay away from them.

Do You Know How The Food Is Prepared?

One thing you need to be very cautious about is how the food is prepared at the junk food restaurants and eateries you love to buy them from. Not all eateries prepare their foods under the best hygienic conditions. Also, some eateries do not know how to minimize the use of certain spices. They add more and more cubes and other spices just to give the food they make the great taste, which makes it unhealthy in the long run.

Cook And Pack For In Lunch Boxes To The Office

Make sure you try your best to cook and pack your food in lunch boxes to work. Doing this helps to save you a lot of money and also helps; you stay stronger as well as feel better.

Make Your Husband Understand Why He Needs To Stay Healthy Through What He Eats

If your spouse loves to eat unhealthy, you can download some stories of other people online and how eating unhealthy affected their lives.

Showing these videos to your husband or spouse will help make them see reason.

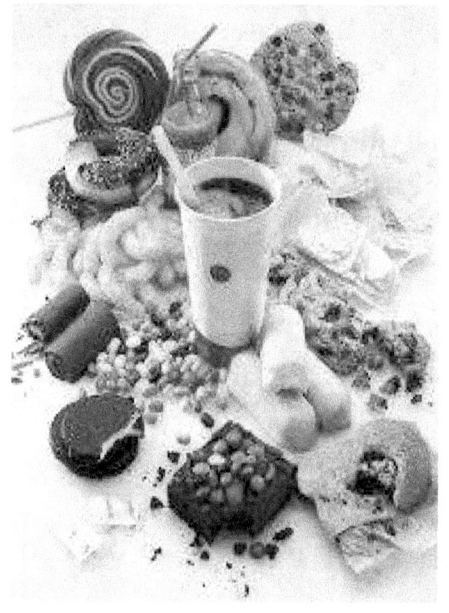

CHAPTER 15
Buy Quality Foods From Online Stores

Make Sure The Online Store Is One You Can Trust

Shopping or buying foods from online stores helps you save a lot of money. Also, when you get a good store, you can buy high-quality foods that will be delivered directly to your home in the perfect condition. However, make sure you buy foods from online stores that have a long standing credibility to offer the best services to their clients.

Do Not Shop For Foodstuffs You Do Not Need

Also, make sure you shop only for foodstuffs you need. Buying foodstuffs you do not need will be a waste of money and time.

Try To Buy Organic Foods

Make sure you buy more organic foods to prevent any negative chemical reaction issues. Organic foods are safe and healthier to eat.

Compare The Prices Of Different Online Stores

Make sure you do not take price for granted. Try you're very best to compare the prices of organic foods from one store to the other. This will help you make the right decision.

Choose Quality Over Quantity

Although saving money is great, it will be better if you stuck to buying quality organic foodstuffs at a reasonable price rather than cheap ones. The probability that cheaper organic foods are truly organic is low. Just make sure you are buying from a credible online store and the rest is history.

FAQ's

- **My son doesn't like broccoli, why should I insist he eats it?**

Broccoli is very healthy and contains lots of nutrients that your son will need to grow better. So, use the two or three bite rule and try to make him love it for his own good.

- **I love honey, but I am afraid my daughters eat it too much.**

Try to have a limit for eating honey. Hide it, but make sure you make it available in lesser quantities when someone needs to eat it. Too much of everything is bad, so get whomever to reduce the amount they consume.

- **How do I get my husband to eat healthily?**

Most men do not take the healthy eating thing seriously till they break down. However, with videos of other victims and the way you go about your eating life, he will be convinced to follow. It takes time, but you will get him to take better care of what he is eating.

- **I love to take health supplements. Is it a better alternative?**

Health supplements are not the sure way out. However, taking them from time to time helps especially if you eat healthily, but are unable to take foods with all vitamins and nutrients you need.

- **My son is not growing the way I want, and I am finding it difficult to make him eat. What do I do?**

Try to get his friends to the house and cook for all of them to try out. This is one way you can get him to eat. Try to lure him into watching movies at the theater, going to the playground, etc.

- **How many times in a day should I eat to stay healthy?**

Eating small quantities of food 3 to 4 times a day helps. Never starve yourself to stay healthy because you will be killing yourself.

- **I am trying to lose weight, but I can't seem to get rid of the junk food. What do I do?**

Just try new recipes at home. You can find healthy recipes with lower calories from the internet.

- **I am a busy woman and do not have much time to cook for myself or my family during the weekdays. What do I do to keep**

the family healthy through eating?

Find time to cook your own meals. The health of your family should be the most important of all for you.

- **My children love to eat toffees and drink a lot of carbonated drinks. Is it healthy for them?**

Canceling it out of their lives will not help. However, you can always reduce their intake of these foods and make them eat healthier and homemade goods.

DISCLAIMER

This Book gives the reader an insight on eating nutritiously to grow well and also how they can stay healthy through the things they eat. It is an original Book with no content copied from any site or book. Therefore, the owner should be contacted if any contents in this book are needed to be used in other books or websites.

The materials written in this Book are unique to this site. The site makes no warranties, uttered, and, therefore, disowns and cancels all other warranties, as well as without restraint, indirect warranties or circumstances of merchantability, or other infringement of rights.

Also, this site does not call for or make any illustrations regarding the precision, probable results, or dependability of the utilization of the materials on this site or if not connecting to such materials or on any websites connected to this website.